I0802178

Aunt Rae's Remedies

Aunt Rae's Remedies

LaRae Olsen

CFI
Springville, Utah

ISBN: 978-1-59955-209-5

Published by CFI, an imprint of Cedar Fort, Inc., 2373 W. 700 S., Springville, UT 84663
Distributed by Cedar Fort, Inc., www.cedarfort.com

Library of Congress Cataloging-in-Publication Data

Olsen, LaRae.
Aunt Rae's remedies / LaRae Olsen.
p. cm.
ISBN 978-1-59955-209-5 (acid-free paper)
1. Home economics. I. Title.

TX158.O57 2008
640--dc22

2008025527

Cover design by Angela Olsen
Cover design © 2008 by Lyle Mortimer
Edited and typeset by Melissa J. Caldwell

Printed in the United States of America

10 9 8 7 6 5 4 3 2 1

Printed on acid-free paper

To a modern pioneer and loving mother
Inez H. White

Contents

Acknowledgments

This is for my mother, Inez White. These are her remedies and a tribute to her life. I would also like to thank Jana Keele, who asked me to write down remedies; Vale White, my first editor; Lanny Olsen, my husband, my sounding board, and my best friend. Also to my writing group for their support—you rock!

Introduction

The village of Teasdale will barely make a dot on any Utah map, but I call it home. Nestled at the base of mighty Boulder Mountain, we the natives were few but were bonded together by common isolation.

We were miles away from the advantages of a large town with a shopping center or medical services. In a real emergency, the chance of getting to a doctor before things got serious was slim. If you were losing lifeblood, you might not make it. Necessity required the people in our secluded region to know and use home remedies.

The one-room country store in our town carried limited provisions. Special orders needed to be placed a week in advance. Therefore, we used household ingredients to make our own soap, home-brewed cough syrup, and bug repellent to make life easier.

In these pages, I will reveal the secret gems of wisdom that I gathered from my childhood.

Cure for Bugs

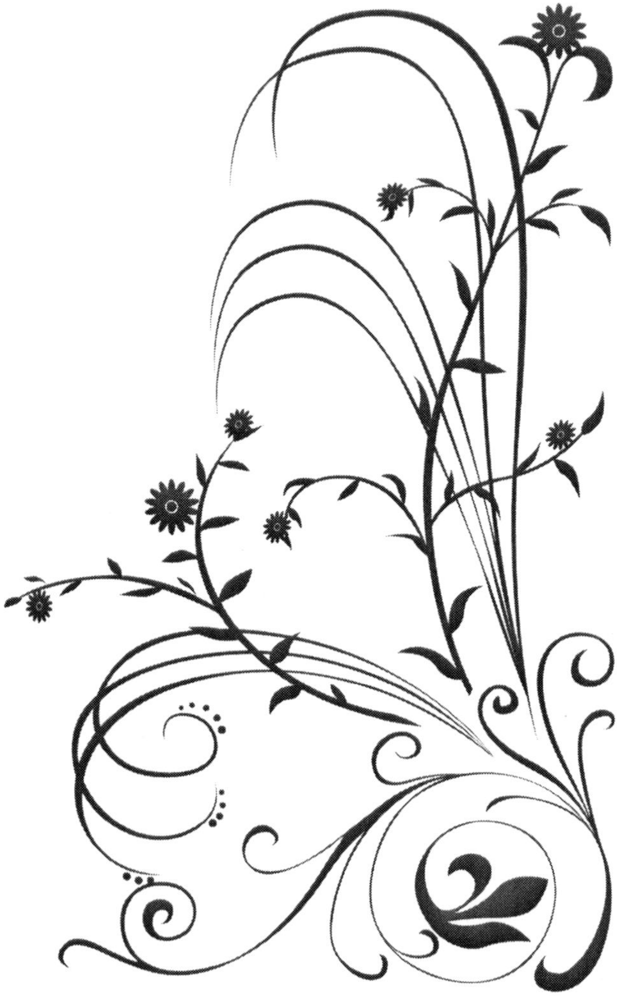

My mother always grew a large garden, a feat she couldn't accomplish without the servitude of her children. We expected, of course, that a large garden would come with a large bug population. Mother's idea of dealing with this infestation was to create a chicken buffet. The kids would fetch the squawking chickens from their coop. All we had to do was open the gate and get out of the way. The fowl flew to their buggy banquet. This generated telephone calls from concerned spectators telling Mom that the chickens were eating her garden. Mom just smiled and said, "That is all right; they're fine."

The poultry did little damage to the plants but would more than make up for it in cheap bug control. In order to escape the massacre, bugs would take refuge in the house.

Well, chickens are not a good idea in the house, so Mother found other ways to get rid of the housebound bugs.

Here are some suggestions to help control these little critters without using poison.

Ants

Although our home was fairly ant-free, we heard a lot of complaints from other neighbors about ants. I found out that Borax works wonders. Borax is a laundry additive found in the soap aisle of most supermarkets. All you need to do is sprinkle a little of the powder around places where the army ants might do their drills. The best place to start is under the sink. Another is under the refrigerator or any cracks where ants could march, like around baseboards.

Borax covers up the chemical trail that ants use to travel from one area to another. Covering up the chemical highway makes it harder for the ants to find their way into your home. Make sure to always sprinkle in places that are away from pets and small children. Although not poisonous, if eaten by a non-ant, Borax could cause a tummy ache or diarrhea.

Bee Stings

Many of the homes in town had an old fashioned front porch where people would gather to visit and gossip. Ours had four large, petrified rocks that stood as sentries and provided solid seats for our visitors. But we also had a bumblebee nest under our front porch, which made a few visits very short.

As a kid I remember sitting in an old red rocker on the porch, watching those bumbling bees come and go. Much to the delight of our resident bumblebees, our lawn was always covered with one of their favorite foods: bright yellow dandelions. This bee activity didn't mix with kids and barefooted summer days.

If you have an unfortunate encounter with the backside of a bee, the first thing you must do (after the screaming stops), is remove the stinger with a clean fingernail or the backside of a pocketknife. Flip the stinger out. Don't try to remove it with tweezers or your fingers. There is a small, microscopic gland at the base of the stinger. Squeezing it will only push more venom into the skin.

Next, pour a little salt into your hand and then add just enough water to make a paste. Dab it on the bee sting and let it dry. You might also try making paste out of meat tenderizer and water. As with the salt paste, apply right to the stung skin. Let this soothing home remedy stay on as long as it will. When it falls off apply an ice pack. This will help to reduce the pain and swelling.

Finally, Kleenex tissues are necessary to wipe away tears.

Roaches

A family member was living in the southern states in a little apartment that had tiny occupants. These pests enjoyed indoor living too. Nights were an adventure—if you had to get up, it was *crunch, squish,* and *pop* all the way to the bathroom.

After a talk with the local tenants, he found that a good roach treatment is boric acid powder. It kills those little creepy bugs without using harsh pesticides. This treatment works because when roaches walk through the boric acid, it collects on their feet and legs. These bugs lick the boric acid off and ingest it. Roaches can't digest the acid. The lethal powder builds up in their digestive system and blocks off any groceries pillaged from your home, so they starve to death.

Sprinkle the boric acid anywhere your resident roaches hide and party, such as under the sink, the bottoms of cupboards, and under the refrigerator.

It takes a bit longer to work than chemical spray, but it is much safer. You need to reapply about every three to six months. Please keep boric acid away from pets, children, and food preparation surfaces. Although borax acid is not a poison, it's not wise to mix the powder with family snacks. You can find boric acid powder in most hardware shops.

Bugs

I have family in Kentucky who worked with valuable horses. The stable owners couldn't use poisons to control bugs around racehorses. An alternate method to make the stable bug-free is to use pepper gas. I'll tell you how to make bug killing gas, but first anything that you don't want dead should be removed from the building. Then make the barn, shed, or house as airtight as possible.

Place a metal pan on a fire-resistant surface. Wad up some newspaper and sprinkle about ½ cup of cayenne pepper powder over the paper. Light the paper on fire and leave immediately. Watch from a window if you must, but be warned, the gas will be strong. The spicier the pepper, the better it works.

To find out just how blistering hot the cayenne pepper is, read the label. It's measured in heat units.

Burning the cayenne powder will make a strong pepper gas that will kill most of the bugs, even in the walls. It does take about two to three hours to work. Once the smoke has subsided, open the doors and windows to air out the area. You may be bothered by the burned odor for a few days, but you won't be bugged anymore.

Biting Flies

A host of blood-sucking insects that thrived in the hot summer weather would torment our old milk cow to the point that she would run through the freshly hung clothes just to get the little pests off her back. Sometimes, in her haste she would rip the clothes off the line and take them with her. The other livestock were not immune to the biting gnats, piercing deer flies, and vicious horse flies.

To help keep peace at the house, and the milk cow out of Mom's laundry, Dad would make a mixture of chewing tobacco and water. He would boil two cups of water and add a can of chewing tobacco (1.2 oz tin) and let it brew overnight. The next morning he would strain the liquid through cheesecloth and pour the smelly mixture into a spray bottle.

He'd apply a heavy mist to the animals' coats and work in. This can be used without harm to the animals, as long as you avoid their eyes. You can reapply as often as needed

The animals welcomed this soothing spray despite the smell, which was preferable to the bloodthirsty insects.

Mosquitoes

Boulder Mountain is full of choice fishing spots, and our family enjoyed this activity. One of my dad's favorite high mountain lakes had a hungry mosquito population. Just as soon as we departed from the truck, they would zero in on our fresh, warm blood supply. New ways needed to be invented to handle this itchy problem.

One way to prevent becoming a lunch buffet for the mosquitoes is to rub garlic juice onto exposed areas of your skin. You won't make any new friends, but this will keep the bloodsuckers at bay for an afternoon. If by chance you encounter a garlic-loving mosquito and he penetrates the juice barrier, try using clear ammonia to relieve the itch. Don't use the ammonia with soap added because this variety might irritate your skin. Just dab a little ammonia on the mosquito's attack site to minimize the itching.

Crushed aspirin mixed with rubbing alcohol works well, too. Just make a paste and apply to the bite. Alcohol helps with the itch, and the aspirin takes the swelling down.

Wasps

One spring I found a tempting, delicate paper wasp nest hanging in our old barn. Wanting to take the nest to school for Show and Tell, I used a long stick and knocked it down. To my amazement, it was full of angry wasps, which proceeded to attack me. I headed at a fast sprint to the back door of the house, screaming at the top of my lungs. Mother opened the door to see who was being murdered.

After getting me safely inside, Mom hunted for something to sooth the pain of the stings. All the while she scolded me for disturbing the nest. She cut a leaf off her aloe vera plant and squeezed out the soothing gel onto the inflamed, red skin. All I had for Show and Tell that week was my bumpy, swollen skin.

Later, I ran onto a remedy in an old magazine for wasp stings. (Sometimes it pays to be a pack rat.) It suggested making a paste of baking soda and water. Apply the paste to the victims of wasp attacks to neutralize most of the poison.

Home Remedies

We woke to about six inches of fresh snow one cold winter morning. It just so happened that was the day my younger brother needed to visit the doctor located over the mountain. It was still early in the morning and the snowplows had not gotten to our town to plow the streets. Needing to get on the road, Mom had to dig our car out because Dad was out of town working. After quite a bit of work shoveling and moving heavy snow, Mom got the car dug out and broke a clear path to the road. Then she went in to get us ready for the trip. While Mom was inside the house, the snowplow came by and buried our car.

When Mom came out and saw what the county boys had done she was fit to be tied—in other words, Mom was mad! With a snow shovel still in hand, she marched over to the general store where the snowplow crew had stopped to get a cup of coffee. She busted in and had a little talk with the boys. Needless to say, the snowplow crew cleared all the snow out of our driveway with a lot of "Yes, ma'am's" in the process.

The moral is "Don't mess with a mad mama."

If Mom had not caught the county boys that day, getting over to the doctor would have been much harder. That's why we depended on home remedies.

Cold Sores

Cold sores have made life miserable for old-timers as well as modern-timers.

My granddad had a strange way of healing cold sores. He would use a small bit of earwax. Yes, that's right, *earwax*. He would take some right from the his ear and put it on the cold sore and press down hard for a few minutes. It would sting and burn a little, but it healed it up right fast. One drawback of this remedy is that you only get a kiss after a lip scrub with major soap and water. This old remedy has been used for generations in my family.

The reason it works is that earwax has antibodies that help kill viruses. When Mom would get a cold sore, she would use this remedy and be rid of her sore in just a few days, while my dad, who thought this remedy was just nasty, would fight his crusty sore for days on end.

Another thing that I have found that works well on a troublesome cold sore is the zinc ointment used in diaper rash creams. I know it might look a little silly putting diaper cream on your lips, but it does work, and it is no worse than earwax. Apply the cream to the cold sore as soon as possible, and keep it on until the outbreak is gone.

Here is a little tip from a country doctor: For a bad cold sore, take a few drops of iodine and paint it right on the sore when it is in the blister stage. Leave it on overnight. This helps kill the virus that causes cold sores. It is important to apply the iodine as soon as the cold sore breaks out. The virus that causes the sore is only active for a short time. You can get iodine at most drugstores, or in the health and beauty aisle at your local market.

Bunions

Those who tamed the rugged West had to walk everywhere they went. So it is not surprising that they had remedies for foot trouble.

Bunions are a painful swelling at the spot where the big toe connects to the foot. Ill-fitting shoes or major foot stress causes them. The older settlers of my hometown used iodine on the trouble spots.

The first thing to do is wash the feet with warm water. Then rub the entire foot down with alcohol to help sterilize. Let it air dry. Paint the iodine right on the bunions. Do this every morning and night until they are gone.

Ice Packs

Bumps and bruises are just part of ordinary farm life. We had many sheds, a barn, and a whole lot of fences to fall off from. The Olympics were aired one summer, and I was fascinated by the girls on the balance beam and wanted to try it. The pasture fence appeared to be a good balance beam.

No, it didn't quite work out that way.

I took a plunge off the fence and hit the hard ground. I was bruised and ran to the house for help. Mom grabbed a bag of frozen vegetables for a quick fix.

The pack wrapped around the boo-boo right nicely. One advantage was that they will stay cold for a long time. Then by evening when the ice pack was no longer needed, supper was half ready.

Heating Packs

Some pioneers used dried-corn heating packs to warm up the bed. They would fill heavy cloth bags with dried field corn and set them by the fire to warm up. When the heating packs were warm, they would place the bag under the cover to take the shock out of a cold bed.

All you need to make a heating pad of your own is some heavy cloth and about three cups of dried corn, beans, or rice. Place the bags into the microwave for one to three minutes; it all depends on the size and speed of your microwave. If you nuke it any longer than three minutes, you might get some funky popcorn.

First Aid Kits

Fishing tackle boxes are not just for fishing anymore. I used one to make a small first aid kit. You can buy any size that you need. All the small compartments can hold many different things. I fill it up with things such as bandages, small scissors, tweezers, and a red washcloth. A red washcloth is the best way to prevent anxiety in younger kids. When kids see blood on a white cloth, they will always panic. Therefore, with the red washcloth, they can't see the blood and that will make the task of cleaning the boo-boo easier. Then apply a magic Band-Aid to speed healing.

Cough Syrup

This very old remedy came from an elderly man that lived in our town. His name was Sam Adams, but most people in town just called him Uncle Sam. He had an opinion on everything and a cure for everything else.

One thing he was famous for was his cough syrup. Taste wasn't one of the qualities of Uncle Sam's cough syrup. One of our neighbors said that when she was a kid she didn't know if it worked or not, but she was so afraid of getting another dose if she continued to cough that she would stop coughing. Before Uncle Sam died, he turned his recipe over to Mom so she could make cough syrup.

Most of all the ingredients you need can be found at the local drug store. Just ask the druggist to help you.

Uncle Sam's Cough Syrup

½ teaspoon Menthol crystals
2 oz. glycerin
½ teaspoon Eucalyptus oil
1 quart Honey
Two tablespoons' good quality whiskey

Mix all ingredients into a large pan and warm very slowly on low heat until mixed well, then store in a cool, dry place in an airtight jar. Use about one tablespoon.

Chicken Pox

When chicken pox would strike, Mom had a fun way of dealing with it. She would take the victim, put them into a tub of warm water, and give them a cold soda pop to drink. This remedy works because chicken pox is a warm temperature-loving bug. The cold soda will make the virus break out as sores on the skin, thus making it a shorter time that you are sick.

It's best to keep very warm after the warm bath because if the virus can retreat back inside the body, then it will make you sicker and will take longer to heal. In dealing with the itching of the pox, use calamine lotion right on the sores. Also, warm baking soda baths will help with the itching.

Cold Soda or Beer Treatment for Cuts

One time our family was out in the mountains gathering a supply of winter wood when an accident occurred. We were cutting a small pine tree down for firewood, and because of a misjudgment, the tree fell on my right shoulder and slid down my arm. I was not hurt badly, but I suffered a long scrape down my arm. We had only a small first aid kit, but no water. My son grabbed a can of cold soda out of the cooler and poured it right on the scrape. I wasn't too happy about losing my soda, but it really got my arm clean. I saw how well it was working so I told him to grab his Dad's soda and pour it over my wound. To the family's surprise, the soda acted like hydrogen peroxide and bubbled out all of the dirt and tree bark. In addition, it was very cold and it helped with the swelling.

When I told a nurse friend of mine about my little discovery, she suggested that a cold beer would work even better because the alcohol in the beer would help fight infection.

Sticky Gum

In the spring when the snow melted and the road to Boulder Mountain became passable, our family would pile into the old pickup truck and head to the hills to gather sticky pine gum. Sticky gum is the yellow sap that gathers on the outside of pine trees in the spring. Mom would give us kids old butter knives and a tin can, and away we would go.

After we got home, Mom took the pine gum and placed it a double boiler. Then she heated the sticky yellow stuff up very slowly. When it melted, Mom skimmed off the dirt and residue. When it cooled a little, she added about a half jar of petroleum jelly. This kept the sticky gum from turning hard again. It was a great salve for infections. Mom always put a small amount on us when she would apply a bandage.

In dealing with sticky gum, we learned a few ways to clean up after it. Take some shortening or butter and add a good amount of salt into the mix. Rub it into the pine gum and wash with warm water.

Cleaning House

Growing up in a large home with a small farm, Mom needed help from us kids to keep things going. We had about a half hour after we got home from school to unwind, change our clothes, and get a snack. After that came the household and farm chores.

Mom had a few fun ways to get the worst jobs done fast. We would draw matches for jobs. Mom would strike one match, let it burn, and blow it out. Then she would put it in her hand with several unlit matches. The burned match was the one we wanted to draw. Whoever got it got first choice of the list of tasks; the winner always chose the easiest job.

Mom taught us how to get a job done fast with cleaning short cuts. Throughout the years, my family has also picked up other cleaning helps. I have listed some of my favorites in this chapter.

Bloodstains

At the hospital where I worked, there were large bottles of hydrogen peroxide in the laundry room. I asked why there was so much peroxide. The staff told me that it was the best way to remove bloodstains. One woman on staff told me that peroxide even worked well on dried and older bloodstains.

After rinsing out as much blood as you can, pour hydrogen peroxide right onto the stain. Let it set for a while and wash as usual. Always check for colorfast on your clothes. I haven't ever had a problem using this little trick.

Permanent Markers

Magic markers and kids always seem to find each other. My sister-in-law told me that she used peroxide to remove marker stains from her kids clothing. I put this advice to the test after finding a large mural drawn on my son's bedroom wall.

I poured undiluted peroxide right on the mark and let it soak in for a while. I rinsed with cool water. It took a few times, but the stain did lift, and painting the room was delayed. Be sure to test it on a small, unseen place so that your wall coverings won't be harmed.

Hard Water Residue

While working in a café in my younger days, I always got stuck with the unpleasant job of cleaning the big coffee pots. The cook showed me a great way to clean off the hard watermarks from the glass pots. She took crushed ice, salt, and vinegar and swished it around in the pot for a short time. The mix removed all of the white hard watermarks. This sure made a hated job a snap to do.

Crayon Remover

Use WD-40 to clean crayon off walls, shoes, and toys. Just spray, let it set for a while, and wipe it clean. I have used the spray on the inside of my dryer when the waxy sticks have been intertwined with the clothes. Unplug the dryer and then spray WD-40 inside and then wipe clean. I have used WD-40 to remove crayon marks from most surfaces that kids covered with their creations.

Therefore, have a few cans of WD-40 for artwork emergencies and make sure that crayons go one drawer higher.

Dishwasher Cleaner

Ever had a bad smell in the dishwasher that will not go away? Something that works well is to pour a cup of vinegar and a handful of salt in your dishwasher and run it on a rinse cycle.

The vinegar and salt remove odor and trapped food that cause a disagreeable odor. The vinegar also removes that white film caused by hard water and the salt cleans the dishwasher on the inside.

Drain Cleaner

Before the day of cholesterol worries, my family used large black cast-iron skillets to fry everything from eggs to steak. The more grease, the better the flavor.

The artery clogging goo would be washed down the drain with the cold dishwater, making grease clogs in the kitchen stink. Mom would put the teakettle on the stove with six cups of water. Then she found the vinegar and baking soda.

Once the water came to a boil, she would pour about a cup of soda into the slow drain. Then she would pour about two cups of the vinegar, followed quickly by the teakettle of hot water. The soda and vinegar would react to clear the drain, and the hot water melted the grease clogs.

Don't worry if it foams up a bit. It's normal for vinegar and soda to do that; it also helps to get any bad smells out of the drain.

Skunk Spray

My brother Wes worked in the hay fields, which unfortunately were also home to a large skunk family. About once a week, their worlds would collide. Wes would be banned to the back porch because of the fumes. Mom would normally use home-canned tomato juice to control the smell.

One day the skunk smell returned and Wes went to the back porch again. Mom made a beeline for the pantry for tomato juice only to find it was gone. Needing something fast, she grabbed a bottle of vinegar and had him use it to get rid of the smell. Acid in the vinegar neutralizes the odor without staining the clothes pink like tomato juice did.

Mom poured one cup of vinegar into the washer and filled it with warm water. She cautiously returned for his pants and shirt from the back porch and dumped them into the machine. It cleaned and deodorized his clothes, so they would be ready for the next skunk encounter.

With this success, she began to experiment with the vinegar to see if it would work on other things. She found that the vinegar treatment would remove skunk smell from all things. People, pets, cars, and even leather goods responds to the vinegar treatment. Use caution when using the vinegar treatment on cats; I still carry the scars.

Ink Stains

My brother Vale had a very tragic accident with his favorite white shirt. A blue ink pen exploded in his pocket, leaving a large, messy ink spot right in the middle of the shirt. His landlord told him to get any cheap hair spray, spray it right on the smudge, and brush hard.

So, this twenty-year-old kid went to the store for hair spray. With a few funny looks from the clerk, he got it. He aimed the spray at the stain and with a little bit of work with an old toothbrush, the ink started to lift. After a few tries and half a can of hair spray later, the stain was gone.

I am happy to report that his shirt did survive.

Homemade Soap

This recipe for homemade soap is from my great-grandmother. It has been handed down through my family. My mother helped make soap with her mother, and I have helped my mother make soap on our back porch. It is a lot of work, but it is a good experience.

Lye soap
5–6 pounds of lard
1 can of lye
1 tablespoon borax
1 cup ammonia
3 pints hot water

Take one pint of the water and add one can of lye to it. Add very slowly and with care. After the lye has dissolved, add the lard and stir well. Add the ammonia, Borax, and the rest of the water. Stir well again. Let it set until it is thick. As the mixture cools, it will set up hard and you can then cut it into bars.

To use homemade soap, take a bar and shave off a few slices with a sharp knife. Add these chips into your washer on the hot water setting and wash as usual. You might want to check to see if all if the soap has dissolved before you rinse. Removed the unused chips of soap and save for later.

Outside Window Cleaner

This is a great window cleaner and a huge time-saver. My kids and I have used this remedy every spring to clean the windows all around the house. It takes about an hour from start to finish.

First remove your screens and spray your windows with a garden hose. Then using the mixture listed below, I always have a child follow this procedure—wash the windows down with a clean sponge mop.

1 gallon hot water
1 tablespoon liquid dish soap
1 cup vinegar
½ bottle liquid Jet Dry

Add all of the ingredients to a large bucket and put a new sponge on your mop. Make sure to close the windows tight. You don't want any water leaks. Take the hose and spray off all dirt from the windows. Scrub the windows with the mop that has been dipped in the bucket of hot water mixture. Rinse the mixture off well with the hose, making sure to get into all of the corners.

Then just walk away. You do not need to worry about wiping dry. The jet dry will sheet off the water and leave a streak-free shine.

Inside Window Cleaner

This window cleaner is a good money saver because it is like the bottled stuff you can buy at the market, but this one is very inexpensive to make. Just for kicks you can add a few drops of blue food coloring so it looks like a famous bottled brand.

1 pint rubbing alcohol
2 tablespoons ammonia
1 tablespoon liquid dish soap
1 gallon water

Mix ingredients well in a large container (I use a clean milk jug). Using a small spray bottle, spray on the windows and clean with a paper towel or soft cloth. When empty, just refill from the larger jug.

Newspaper for Windows

As a teenager, I would help the women in our small town with their spring-cleaning. This was a good way for a young girl to make some extra pocket change. One older lady was very fussy about her windows. I had to use newspaper to buff dry all of the windows and mirrors in her house. She told me that it was the printers' ink in the paper that made the windows shine so beautifully. She was right because she had the best-looking windows in town. Using the old newspaper will also help in reducing that pile of newspapers in your garage.

Mini Blinds

Mini blinds were all the rage just a few years ago. I fell victim to the fad and had to have a set of my own. Sadly, I found that dust bunnies love them too. Spring cleaning arrived and those blinds needed a cleaning.

I filled the tub with hot, soapy water and dropped the blinds in, dust bunnies and all. I dunked them up and down a few times to remove stubborn dirt. Then I rinsed in cool water with a few drops of Jet Dry (a rinsing agent) and they dried spot-free. This also helps to keep them bunny free.

Personal Care

The old house that I grew up in did not have a modern water heater until I was in grade school. Mom would build a fire in the wood-burning stove that had what was known as water jackets. The water ran through pipes into the fire box of the stove and back to a water tank. The water would heat up when there was a fire. On Saturday morning Mom would build a fire to heat the water for Saturday night baths.

The tradition was that Dad would go first, then Mom, and followed by the kids, oldest to the youngest. This is where the expression "Don't throw the baby out with the bathwater" came from.

I love to take long baths with some scented oils and soft candlelight. I have been known to take a bath any time of the day, from midnight to noon. It is my hideaway from stress and life's pressures. That's why I offer my hideaway bath salt recipe first, for your reading and relaxing pleasure.

BATH SALTS

My first home had an old-fashioned cast iron claw-footed tub. It was deep enough to submerge yourself into the silky depths of hot water. The bathtub would hold the heat for a long time. I would make my own bath salt, take a book, and spend the afternoon in the tub.

Nice fantasy, but in truth it was just a few stolen minutes away from the kids, dogs, and phone ringing. However, this bath salt makes those few minutes well worth it.

1 cup rock salt
1 cup baking soda
1 tablespoon mineral oil
1 tablespoon scented oil
10 drops food coloring (optional)

Mix well in a large bowl. Make sure that all of the ingredients are well blended. It will take a little stirring to completely mix the salt and oil. You can find great scented oils at your local craft store in the candle department. After you get the mixing done, just add about two tablespoons of bath salts to a tub of warm water, and don't forget the candles.

Just a hint: don't use yellow food coloring—it will turn the water a questionable yellow color.

Bath Powder

The Boy Scout troop from my hometown was working on a 50-Miler Afoot/Afloat Award.

To earn this award, the troop had to hike fifty miles, down the backside of the Boulder Mountain to the shores of Lake Powell. Leaving town with large backpacks and a great amount of courage, they headed across the rough country for a six-day outing.

Mom packed a box of cornstarch in my brother's backpack to help prevent chafing. It works as well as bath powder and has no girly scent that would repulse any self-respecting Boy Scout. When the other scouts found out about his secret cornstarch stash and how well it worked, it was raided. He almost ran out before they got to their destination.

If you want a flowery scent, take one-cup cornstarch and add 5-6 drops of scented oil. These oils are available in the potpourri and candle department of most stores.

Mix well in a plastic bag and then store in an air-tight jar. It is a great after-bath powder. With all of the scented oil on the market, you can experiment for your own unique fragrance.

Hair Rinse

My mom had the softest, shiniest chestnut brown hair that cascaded in waves down her back. Mom spent hours putting her hair up in bobby pins that would create the waves. To keep her hair in great shape, she never used anything but a good generic shampoo followed by a vinegar rinse, which would clean off soap residue.

I use it to this day, and it works wonderfully except the slight smell of vinegar, which reminded me of my mother's vinegar and oil salad dressing.

My sister Sherma found out that lemon juice would remove soap reside, too. Therefore, we started to use lemon juice because a teenage girl would rather smell like lemons than walking salad dressing.

To get your hair clean and glossy, shampoo your hair, then rinse out the shampoo. Mix equal parts of vinegar and warm water. Slowly pour the mixture over your hair, working it in. Rinse it out with cool water, and style as usual.

Untangling Kids' Hair

The day care center where my kids were enrolled had a great method of dealing with tangles in little girls' hair. The women at the center would make a game of it.

They would escort the girls to the pretend beauty shop in the back of the center. There was a special place set up with a little stool and a table with the combs and hair pretties in cute little jars. The staff would take a spray bottle of warm water and add about one tablespoon of hair conditioner, shaking it well in the spray bottle Then they would spray the mixture into the little girls' hair, working it into the tangles.

By offering their own beauty shop for the little girls, the staff provided a fun way to get styled hair. Hair conditioner is cheap and so is a spray bottle, so you can polish your little princess as easily as the professionals can.

Toothpaste

After we finished supper and the dishes were washed, it was time to brush our teeth and get ready for bed. One night this routine ground to a squelching halt. We were out of toothpaste, and the store was closed until Monday morning. Dad had us use a concoction from his childhood. He mixed up baking soda and salt, and then we dipped our toothbrush into the mixture. Hurriedly we brushed our teeth. It was far from mint fresh, and we had the look of a rabid dog, but the baking soda freshened our breath and the salt polished our teeth.

I was glad Dad was not as old as the pioneers because their solution was outlandish. They would use a strange combination of ingredients to clean their teeth—charcoal and honey. They pulverized the charcoal into a fine powder and then mixed it with honey. It kept the teeth very white and helped to prevent tooth decay and gum diseases.

Hair Gel

One Halloween my kids wanted to dress up as punk rockers with wild clothes and stiff, spiked hair. At the local thrift store, we got supplied with the wild clothes, but the spiked hair was a trouble spot. We tried hair spray, but we needed something stronger to hold the hair into the desired spikes. A friend suggested using hair gel. She told us that she made her own out of gelatin and hot water. We were off to the kitchen to make hair gel. We took two packages of the Knox brand gelatin and let them dissolve into a cup of boiling water. When it cooled, we spiked the kids' hair, and they were off for a fun-filled night of begging for candy and catching donuts on the spikes.

Dealing with Emergencies

In my hometown at least one day a month, the power would go out and leave us without electricity for hours, sometimes even days.

One cold Saturday night the power went out because of a snowstorm. By morning, the temperature dropped to below zero. Mom got up Sunday morning, built a large fire in the wood burning stove, and started cooking breakfast. When her family was fed, they were banished to the bitter cold to get the chores done. Mom called the neighbors to come over and get warm and fed.

That Sunday, church was held in the welcoming shelter of my mother's warm kitchen.

Oil Lamps

Nothing brings back my childhood memories faster than the smell of a burning oil lamp. There's just something about that unique smell and the soft light a lamp puts out that is special to me. On nights that the electric power was down, Mom would set a coal oil lamp in the middle of the kitchen table, and we kids could do our homework while Mom cooked supper on the woodburning stove.

You can still buy these lamps at furniture or hardware stores. They come in many styles, and now you can get various kinds of scented oils that are much nicer than kerosene.

The lamps would come in three parts—the base, the wick assembly, and the chimney. The base is the bottom part that is filled with oil. The wick and the base come apart so you can fill the base. The wick needs to be trimmed, so it doesn't put out to much smoke. You do this by cutting the corners off the wick forming a point. Replace the wick into the base of oil. The wick needs to have time to soak up the oil, so let it sit for a short time. The chimney is the glass top, which clips into the wick piece.

Don't wait for power to go out to light your lamps. Hit the breaker box, turn off the electricity, and have a pioneer appreciation night. See just how ready you are for emergencies.

Outdoor Refrigerator

In 1965 there was a big flood that hit our little town. The incredible force of the unrelenting water took out the light pole by our house and plunged us into total refrigeratorless-ness.

The dark water spread and ate up the land between the world and our home. With the power out and no way to know when it would be back on, panic was upon us because we had two refrigerators full of food and no way to keep them cold.

Mom knew what to do. She told us to haul the contents of the refrigerators outside and put them into wooden milk crates. Thinking that she had lost it, we did as she asked. Then she draped burlap over the boxes, looped our hose over the top, and let a small trickle of water soak the burlap. She explained to us wide-eyed children that this makes an evaporated cooler for the food.

The food inside kept cool enough not to spoil for days. Something else that works great for a backup is a picnic cooler.

Emergency Candles

Our small Cub Scout troop consisted of four little boys that were the terror of the town. The Scoutmaster needed a project to keep these little rabble-rousers out of mischief. He couldn't have dreamed up a worst horror for them than tuna fish can candles.

My brother Vale hated tuna fish and normally refused to eat it in any form. However, the Cub Scouts force-fed him tuna fish so they could have enough cans to make the candles.

Take an old cardboard box and cut a strip just as wide as the can and about two feet long. Roll it very tightly and place it in the tuna can. Pour melted wax right into the tube until filled. Pull the very center of the cardboard up just a bit to use as a wick.

Whether you love or hate tuna fish, you can make candles of your own, and this one is dolphin approved.

Sunburns

In the late 1960s we didn't have the information that too much sun causes skin cancer. So on the first warm spring day, all the girls would take the sleeping bags out and throw them on to the almost frozen ground, to get a start on the great summer tan. However, most of the time all we got was a very bad sunburn. After a day of foolish sun worship, our skin was on fire.

To cool the fire of the sunburn, we got the vinegar treatment. Pour vinegar into your hand, place it right onto the burned skin, and get out of the way—it stings! However, in a few minutes, the stinging will stop, and some of the heat will be gone. Aloe vera gel will take out the rest of the burn and also keep the skin from drying out.

If you don't have an aloe plant, get one. The fresh gel works great for many cut and burns. We used aspirin to help with the swelling but with the latest news about aspirin, you might want to use one of the aspirin substitutes.

Bumps

One afternoon I was visiting with a friend when her one-year-old daughter fell and hit her mouth on the edge of a coffee table. Surprise registered on the baby's face, and then a long howl started that I am sure only a dog could hear. My friend panicked at the sight of blood and the swelling lip. Unsure how to stop the dogs and the child from howling, she turned to me for help. I grabbed the baby's bottle and filled it with cold water. The child took it, and in a few minutes, the screaming stopped, our ears returned to normal, and the dogs went to sleep. The cold water had reduced the swelling, and the bottle had quieted the toddler.

Mustard Plaster

Lying on the couch watching cartoons was a first-rate way to spend Saturday morning. If you had a chest cold and were all stuffed up, the cartoons lost some of their appeal. One cold Saturday morning, I was congested, coughing, hacking, and suffering on the couch. Mom came in with an old remedy that Grandmother had used on her. Good old mustard plaster. Embarrassing as it was to have a mixture of yellow goo all over my chest, the concoction warmed my skin and started breaking up the tightness in my lungs, and I could breathe easier.

This is a very old chest cold remedy:

5 tablespoons of flour
3 tablespoons of vegetable oil
1½ teaspoon of dry powdered mustard
Enough warm water to make a paste

Mix all the ingredients into the warm water until it makes a thick paste. Spread it over a clean cotton cloth or cheesecloth. Fold the cloth over and place it on the chest. (Don't place the paste right on the chest because it might burn.) Leave it on for about five to ten minutes but check it often. If there is any redness, remove immediately. After a time remove the cloth and wipe off all residue with a warm cloth. Rub the chest lightly with Vicks.

Alcohol wrap

As with most households, we had our share of sore throats. It seems that whenever you have a cold, a cough always keep you up at night. Mom would soak an old rag in rubbing alcohol, and then wrap it around the sufferer's neck and send them off to bed. As we settled into our pillows, our throats cooled and sleep came at last.

This is an old remedy that was used by my great-grandmother. I used it for my own kids, and it got them through some rough nights.

Now don't go out and buy some medicinal Jack Daniels for this treatment! Remember, it was rubbing alcohol we used.

Ice in a Swamp Cooler

One hot summer day I had a call from Las Vegas; my brother was on the line complaining that it was over 120 degrees in the shade and getting hotter. His swamp cooler was just not keeping the place cool at all.

I suggested that he go out, buy some blocks of ice, and put them into the swamp cooler.

Later that night he called back and told me that I had turned him into an ice addict. Now he had to buy ice for the cooler because it had worked so well. His place was almost too cold.

I started knitting a scarf with matching mittens.

Doggie Lambs Care

On our little farm were many kinds of animals that needed care. Most of them turned into pets. Mom would round up doggie (motherless) lambs from the local sheep rancher. These lambs would be in bad shape. They were rejected by their mothers and often had been kicked and trampled by the herd. Mom had to work fast to warm them up and get them fed. She made a formula of canned milk and eggs to feed the little lambs. The lambs had to be fed about ever two or three hours, so Mom would get up and feed them, just like a mother with a new baby. One year she took her little pets to the market to sell them. Because of her loving care, the sheep topped the market and took the highest price of the day.

Bloated Cattle

When I was a just a youngster, one of our milk cows had gotten into the grain and was bloated. This is when cows eat too much rich grain or real leafy hay, and they get excess gas in their stomachs. Since a cow has more than one stomach, it is hard for them to release the trapped gas. The expanding stomachs crowds their lungs to the point that the animal suffocates. Without some quick help, our milk cow would have died. Since dad was out of town and was not around to help and she wasn't sure what to do, my mom called Granddad Hunt. He remembered an old remedy. He told my mom to take a large handful of cayenne pepper and rub it all over the cow's mouth and tongue, making sure to get as much as she could inside the cow's mouth. He explained that the cow would fight to get the pepper off its tongue and by doing so, the tongue would drop and the mouth could open wide enough to release most of the gas.

So, with flashlights in hand, we headed to the barn to save our cow. We moved the cow into the stable and gave her the dose of the cayenne pepper, just as Granddad told us. After a few tense moments, the old cow let out a giant belch and released the trapped gas. With a sigh of relief from all of us, the cow was soon better.

Today, I tell cattlemen about this remedy and they always give me a laugh. If they had been in our barn that night, they would have tried it for themselves.

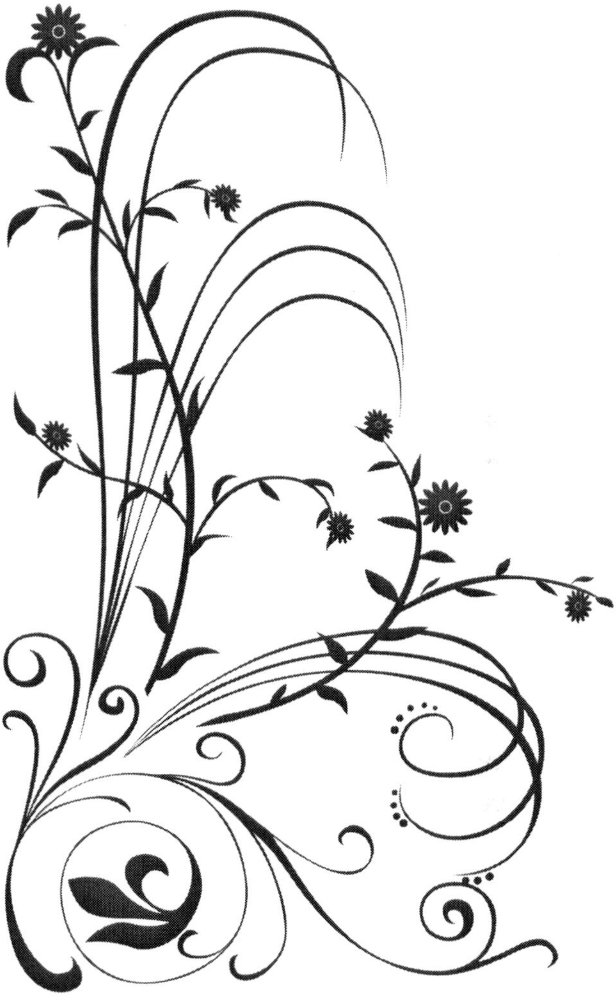

GARDENING

In earlier days everyone had a kitchen garden. In these gardens, they would raise most of the vegetables for their family to use in the wintertime. The produce was bottled, dried, or frozen.

Like most households in our area, we too had our kitchen garden. But unlike most people, Mom's garden covered close to a third of an acre. Almost every kind of garden vegetable that you could think of was there. Corn, beans, squash, and many other vegetables were grown and put away for the winter. Part of the vegetables were stored in what was known as the "tater pit." It was a dark, cool root cellar that was at the bottom of the garden, and it kept the food good all winter. Potatoes and carrots were put into the pit and covered with a layer of straw.

Mom found a way to keep apples in the pit, too. The apples were picked and each one was wrapped in a piece of newspaper and placed into a box. Then the box was put into the cellar

Pumpkin pie is a Thanksgiving tradition, but once you have had warm apple pie from apples that you have grown and stored yourself, you will change that tradition.

Vegetables as Flowers

For our hard work and getting our 4-H club project done on time, our leaders took us to the Utah State Fair. After a four-hour bus ride, we arrived in the big city. We unloaded at the front of the exhibition building and were shocked to find that there were vegetables growing in all of the flower beds. The local 4-H club had planted all kinds of vegetables in the flower beds. It looked very festive, and you could eat them, too. Smaller plants, like carrots, were used as borders, and taller plants, like tomatoes, peppers, and onions, were used in the back. Squash plants, cucumbers, and pumpkins were planted as ground cover.

No matter what you grow, whether you are trying for a blue ribbon or just something fresh for the dinner table, remember, if you can grow flowers, you can grow vegetables.

Composting

Cleaning out the cow barn was just a nasty job that needed to be done. The manure was scooped up with a shovel and thrown out into the corral. In the springtime, the pile was hauled out and spread on the garden. Not knowing that we were composting at the time, we just knew that this step was needed to grow happy vegetables.

Not too many cows can be found in neighborhoods today, but there are still ways to get good soil by composting yard waste. Use all of your leaves on your garden and flower beds. Rake them in the fall onto the beds and then in the spring turn the soil under before you plant the seedling. They make the soil loose and help hold the water better around the plants. Leaves, newspaper, and shredded paper all make great composting material.

So start shedding those endless credit card applications and turn them into great tasting summer dinner.

Onions against Bugs

Early in the spring, Mom would plant tomato seeds onto boxes of soil and place them in our "hot house," a south-facing shed that sat at the bottom of the garden. When the danger of frost had past, the tender plants were replanted into the garden. Mom would plant an onion bulb between each tomato, cabbage, and pepper plant. The stout smell of the onion would turn away the nasty plant predators.

Flowers have been used to repel bugs, too. Marigolds have a strong fragrance that can be used to keep bugs off garden plants, and they look pretty, too.

Tomatoes in Straw Bales

After watching a TV show on gardening, my husband got a great idea. He planted our tomatoes into straw bales. Along the south side of our house were lines of straw bales with little green plants peeking out.

If you have limited room and would like to try this, go to the local pet supply place and buy some bales of straw. With a sharp knife, cut a six-inch diameter that's about six inches deep and fill with potting soil. Plant the tomatoes and pack the soil around them good and tight. After some tender loving care, you will have fresh tomatoes.

About the Author

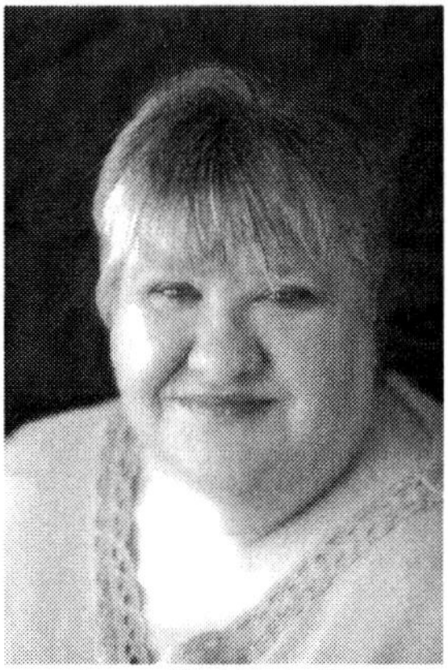

Courtesy of Nick Marsing Photography
Manti, Utah

LaRae Olsen grew up in Teasdale, Utah, set in the beautiful heart of Wayne County. At the feet of her mother, Inez White, she learned how to use remedies to heal family members and farm animals alike. By request from friends, she began to write down cures she remembered using as a child and placed them in her mother's old tin box. Ten years and many rewrites later, her book was finally finished.

LaRae now lives in central Utah with her husband, Lanny. They have three children, Jennifer, Brandon, and Karen. LaRae worked for the local newspaper as a Senior Style columnist and is involved with a writing group that has been a great resource and support to her talent.

0 26575 52095 8